DATE DUE			
SE 21 '95			

KI

LF

LP

THE BURIED BODY

USA

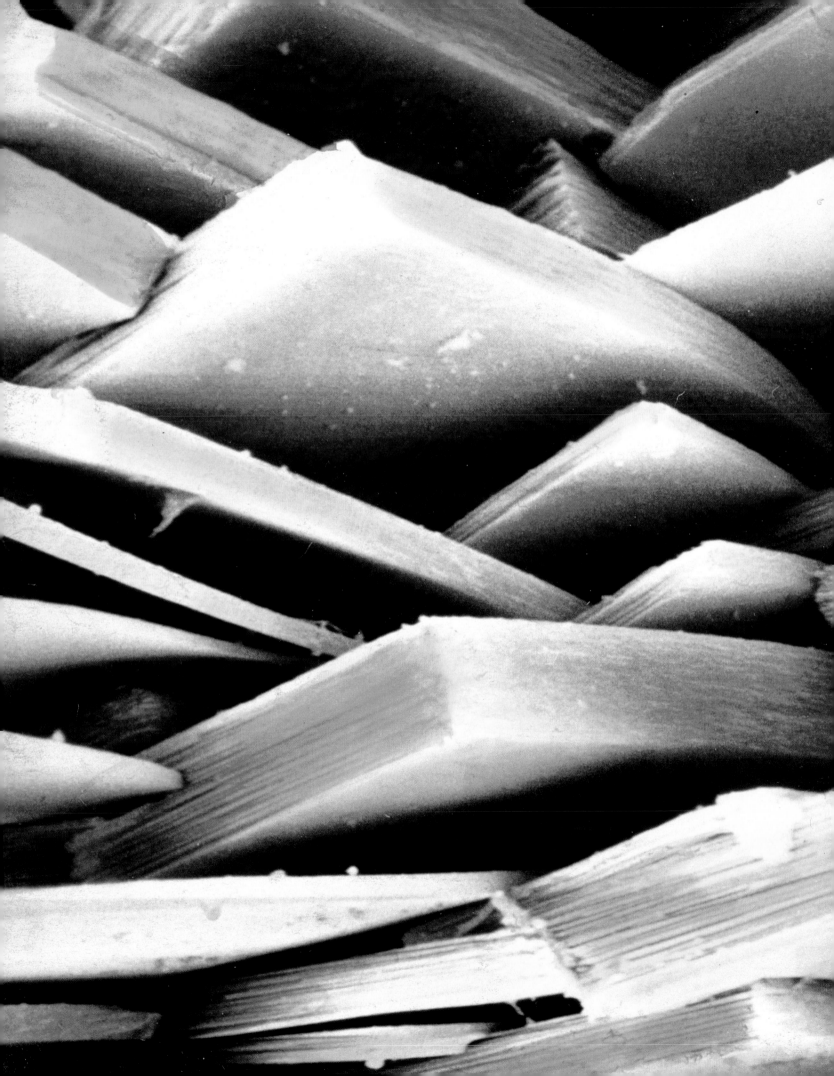

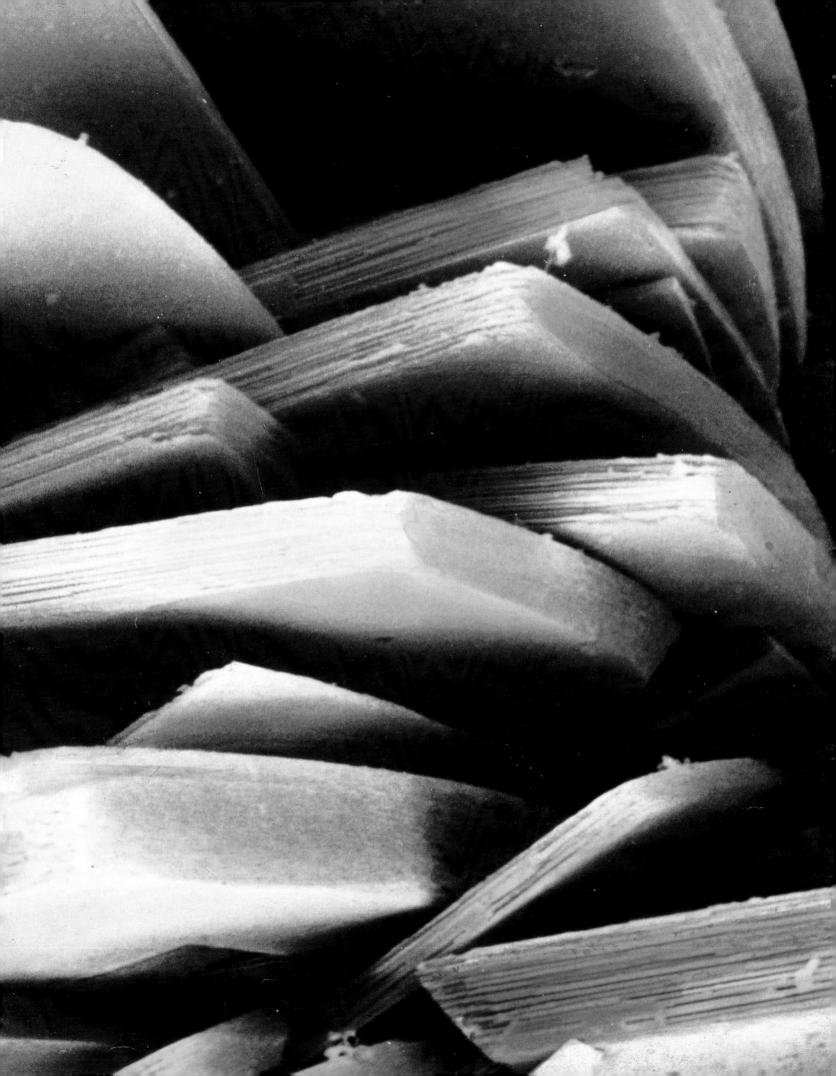

DISCOVER HIDDEN WORLDS

THE
HUMAN BODY

By Heather Amery and Jane Songi

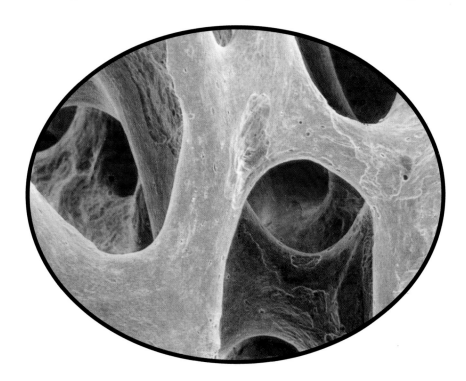

A GOLDEN BOOK · NEW YORK

Western Publishing Company, Inc., Racine, Wisconsin 53404
Printed in Italy

CONTENTS

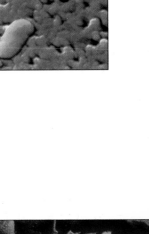

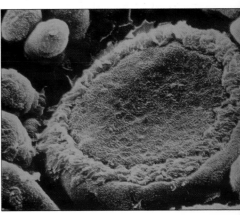

INTRODUCTION

Look closely at the world around you. All sorts of small things you might never have noticed before—a grain of sugar, a tiny insect, a speck of dust—may come into view. And if you use a magnifying glass, you will surely see even more.

Microscopes that use light and have several glass magnifying lenses were invented nearly 400 years ago. For the first time, scientists could see the germs that cause disease, the countless cells in our blood, and millions of other things that no one knew existed. Modern light-using microscopes can magnify an object up to 1,000 times its normal size.

We can look even more closely at the world with electron microscopes, which were invented about 60 years ago. Instead of using light, electron microscopes use a beam of electrons to "look" at tiny things, magnifying them up to 200,000 times.

In this book you will see parts of the human body—plus a few other things—greatly magnified. From the ends of your hair to the tips of your toes, the human body is brought into vivid focus. Color has been added to enhance some of the items shown.

Magnifications in this book are generally given beneath the pictures and consist of a multiplication sign followed by a number. For example, x 25 means that the object is shown at 25 times its actual size. Where there is no magnification given, the photo is simply an enlargement.

▲ The researcher above is using an electron microscope to examine a tiny object. The magnified pictures show up on a television screen.

▼ The technician below is using a light microscope to study samples of bacteria.

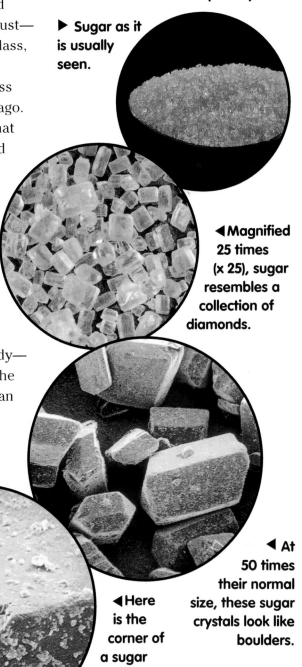

▼ Look closely at a spoonful of sugar, and you can see that each grain is a roughly shaped crystal.

▶ Sugar as it is usually seen.

◀ Magnified 25 times (x 25), sugar resembles a collection of diamonds.

◀ At 50 times their normal size, these sugar crystals look like boulders.

◀ Here is the corner of a sugar crystal magnified 500 times.

AT YOUR FINGERTIPS

What would you do if your hands suddenly disappeared? You wouldn't be able to hold a book or dial a telephone or catch a ball or draw a picture. Your hands are extremely sensitive, and without them your contact with the world would be greatly diminished. The numerous nerve endings that are in your fingers send messages to your brain and allow you to feel things that are rough or smooth as well as hot or cold. To protect the delicate tissue below, the skin on your palms is tough and thick—tougher and thicker, in fact, than the skin anywhere else on your body except the soles of your feet.

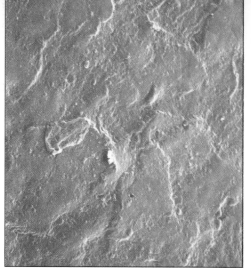

Surface of nail
(x 300)

Personal prints

Look at your fingertips. The patterns of small loops on them are your fingerprints, and they are different from almost everyone else's. The chance that two people will have the same prints is about 1 to 64 billion. To take your own fingerprints, dab your fingers in ink or paint and press them onto paper.

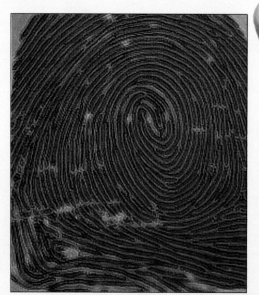

Fingerprint

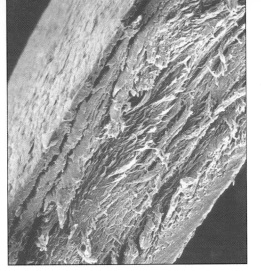

End of nail
(x 100)

◀ **Tough as nails.** Your nails protect your fingers and toes from bumps and blows that could damage the ends. Nails grow all the time, but slowly—less than 1/10 of an inch a month. If you lose a nail, it would take about six months to grow it back.

Nails are made of a tough substance called keratin, the same thing your hair is made of. The reason cutting your nails doesn't hurt is that the nail itself is dead. The "half moons" on your nails look white because of air pockets where the nails are joined to the skin underneath.

▼ **People lose skin all the time as little flakes fall off or are rubbed off. During your life, you will shed about 40 pounds of skin.**

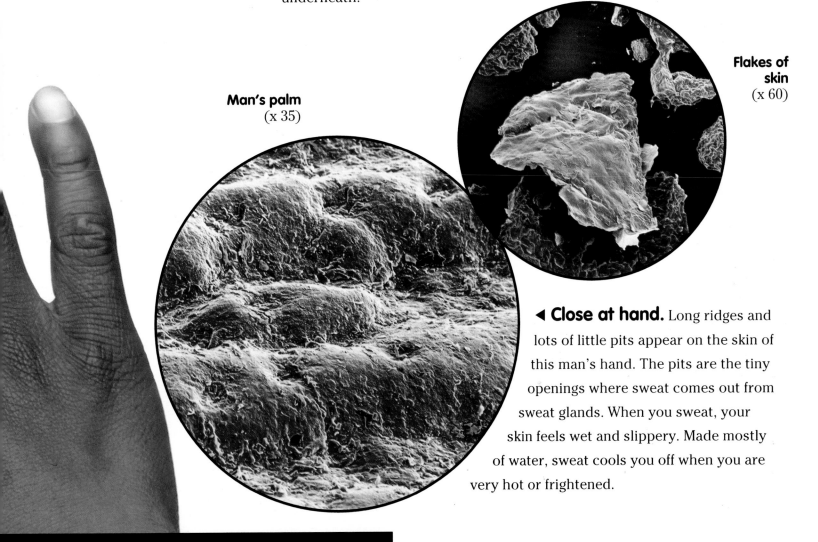

Man's palm
(x 35)

Flakes of skin
(x 60)

◀ **Close at hand.** Long ridges and lots of little pits appear on the skin of this man's hand. The pits are the tiny openings where sweat comes out from sweat glands. When you sweat, your skin feels wet and slippery. Made mostly of water, sweat cools you off when you are very hot or frightened.

A MAN IN INDIA HAD A THUMBNAIL THAT WAS OVER **45** INCHES LONG — MORE THAN THREE TIMES THE HEIGHT OF THIS PAGE!

Skin Deep

Skin, your body's largest organ, is a tough, waterproof cushion and a barrier against disease-carrying germs. It protects your inner organs and also works as a kind of thermostat, helping to keep you at the right temperature. In sunlight, skin can even make vitamin D, one of the vitamins we need to stay healthy.

▼ **Under your skin.** Skin gets its color partly from blood vessels. When you are hot, the blood vessels get bigger, letting more blood through. This helps you shed heat and makes you look red. When you are cold, the blood vessels get smaller, and the amount of blood in them decreases. This makes you look paler. It also helps prevent heat loss from your body. The nerve endings in your skin are sensitive to heat, cold, touch, pressure, and pain. Pain helps to keep your body healthy by signaling you when you are injured or sick.

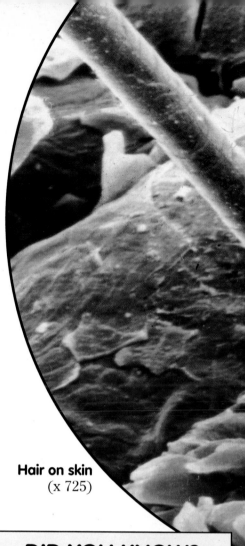

Hair on skin
(x 725)

DID YOU KNOW?

On a warm day, an adult male loses about a quart of sweat—enough to fill a milk carton. On a really hot day, he may lose up to 8 quarts of sweat! This makes him very thirsty, and his body needs extra salt to make up for the salt lost in the sweat.

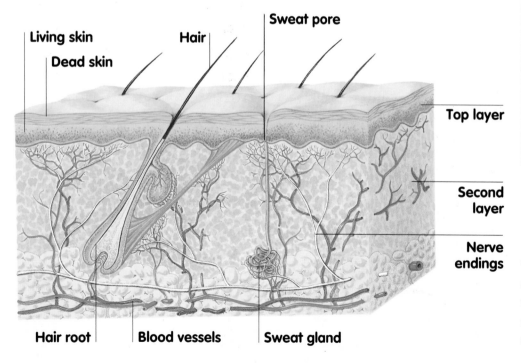

Living skin
Dead skin
Hair
Sweat pore
Top layer
Second layer
Nerve endings
Hair root
Blood vessels
Sweat gland

◄ Skin has two main layers. The top layer sheds flakes of old, dead skin while new skin grows underneath. In the second layer are sweat and oil glands, as well as the roots of hair and nails.

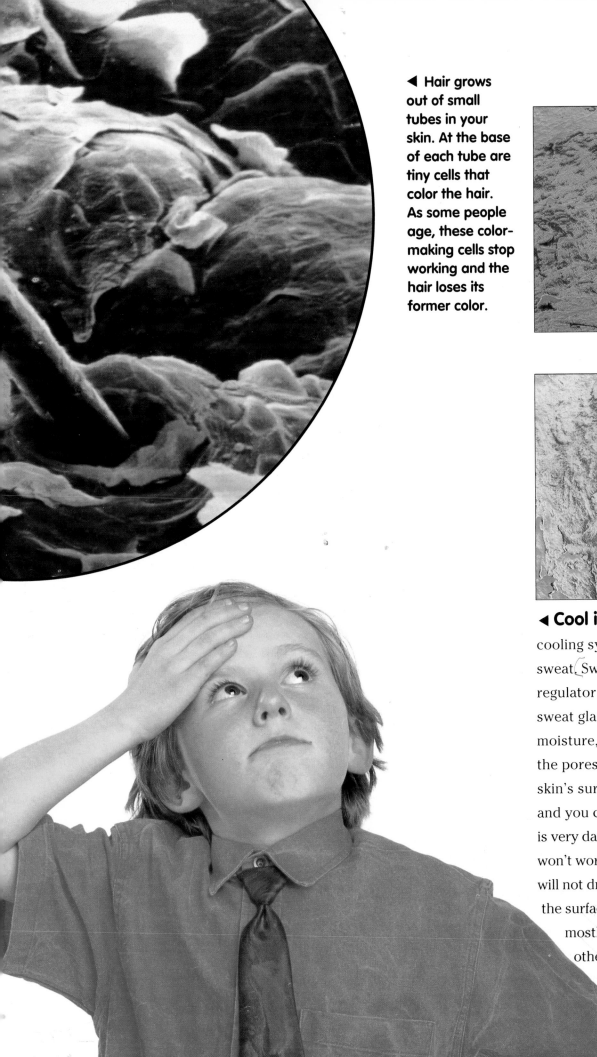

◄ Hair grows out of small tubes in your skin. At the base of each tube are tiny cells that color the hair. As some people age, these color-making cells stop working and the hair loses its former color.

Sweat pores in skin
(x 150)

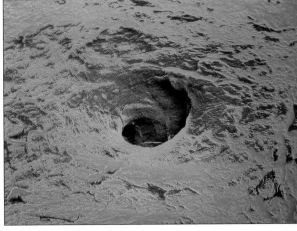

(x 260)

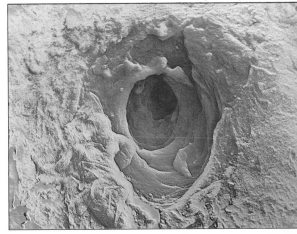

◄ **Cool it.** Just as buildings have cooling systems, the body has sweat. Sweat is your temperature regulator. When you get very hot, sweat glands in the skin produce moisture, which is released through the pores. As the sweat dries on the skin's surface, the heat is removed and you cool off. If the air around you is very damp, your cooling system won't work as well because the sweat will not dry as quickly when it reaches the surface of your skin. Sweat is mostly water with some salt and other chemicals in it.

Hairs by the Hundreds

There's no doubt about it: People are just plain hairy. You have hair growing out of the skin on almost every part of your body except your lips, the palms of your hands and soles of your feet, and the sides and tips of your fingers and toes. Some hair, like the hair on your head, is thick and can easily be seen and felt. Other hair, like the hair on your earlobes, is so fine and short that it can't be seen unless you look very closely. You inherit the color and texture of your hair from your parents. Altogether, you have about 5 million hairs growing on your body or falling out all the time.

New hairs
(x 185)

◄ **Three-year cycle.** The average hair on a person's head grows about three years before it falls out. If hair is not cut regularly or is bleached or dyed, the ends of the hair may become unhealthy and frayed. The end of the hair on the left is ragged and split.

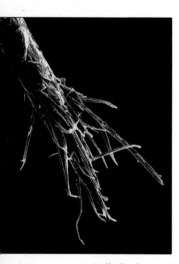

Split hair end
(x 400)

Hair root
(x 170)

MOST PEOPLE HAVE BETWEEN 100,000 AND 200,000 HAIRS ON THEIR HEAD.

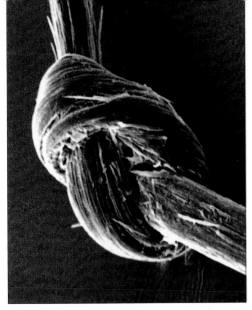

◀ When a strand of hair gets tiny knots in it, the surface becomes rough, and short pieces begin to break off. A normal, healthy head of hair has long, smooth strands. Each hair is hollow and coated with keratin—the same tough material your nails are made of.

Knotted hair
(x 300)

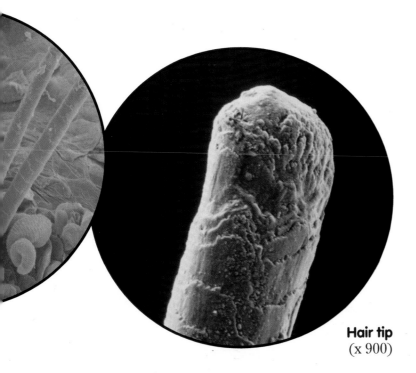

Hair tip
(x 900)

▲ **A hair-raising episode.** In the "new hairs" close-up above, three hairs can be seen growing out of a person's head. The short fat one is brand-new. The two thinner ones are older. Under the skin, each hair has a root and a very small gland that supplies the hair with oil to make it smooth and glossy. Every hair also has a tiny muscle that pulls it upright when a person is scared or cold—making it seem to "stand on end."

Normal hair
(x 475)

CUTTING BACK

Hair is dead—or at least the part you can see is dead. The root, which is the living part of the hair, is under your skin. It hurts when your hair is pulled because your roots are being tugged. A haircut won't hurt, but plucking out a hair with tweezers will, since you are pulling the live part out of your skin.

▼ **A close shave.** The hair on most men's faces grows a little every day, but some men shave it off. They use razors with shaving cream and water or electric shavers. Below are close-ups of the hair shaved from a man's chin. An electric razor cuts the hair into ragged sections. A sharp razor blade usually slices off the hair in neater pieces.

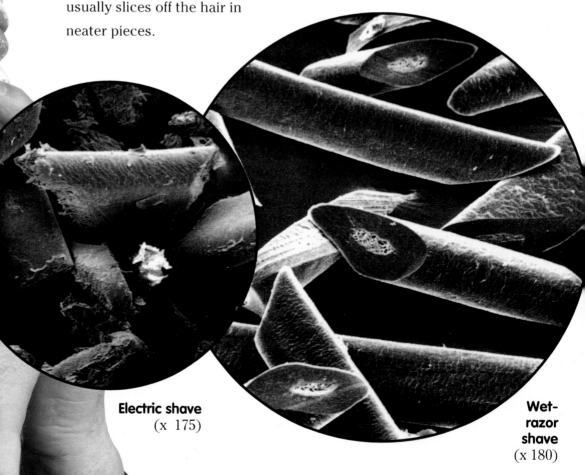

Electric shave
(x 175)

Wet-
razor
shave
(x 180)

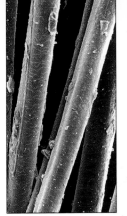

Dirty hair
(x 80)

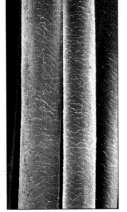

Clean hair
(x 80)

▲ Hair on your head gets dirty very quickly. The hair shown here was washed four days before this photograph was taken. You can see it is already coated with tiny particles of dead skin and dust.

▲ This hair has just been shampooed and is smooth and particle free.

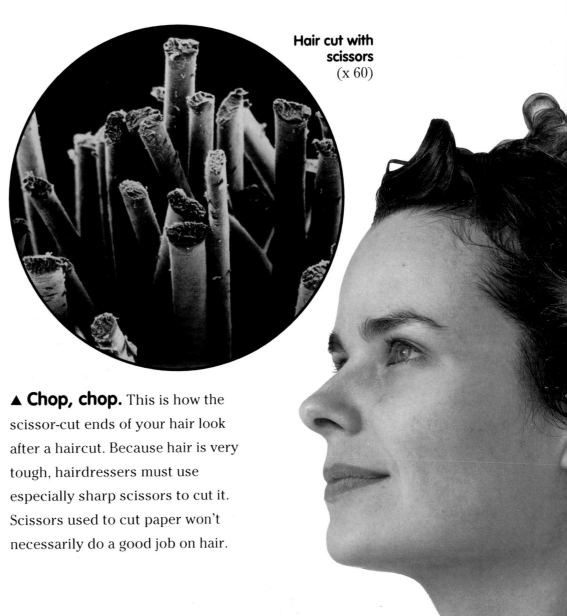

Hair cut with scissors
(x 60)

▲ **Chop, chop.** This is how the scissor-cut ends of your hair look after a haircut. Because hair is very tough, hairdressers must use especially sharp scissors to cut it. Scissors used to cut paper won't necessarily do a good job on hair.

Sticky spray

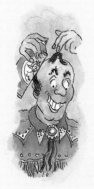

Hair spray is a type of lacquer, or varnish, that people spray on their hair to keep the hairs neatly in place or "set" in a particular style. The spray comes out in tiny drops and dries very quickly, coating the hairs and making them stick together.

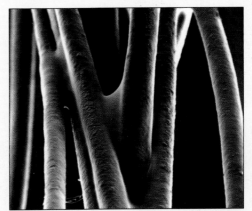

Hair spray on hair
(x 130)

A QUESTION OF TASTE

When you say something tastes good, you are usually talking about food that you've put into your mouth. But your nose helps you to taste, too. Usually you smell something before you eat it. Smelling food gives you a clue as to what it will taste like. The smell of good food also makes your mouth water. The saliva, or spit, in your mouth helps you to digest your food as you chew it. Even when the food is in your mouth, your nose still has a role in helping you to taste it.

Odor-sensitive skin
(x 15,500)

Odor-sensitive skin

Nostrils

Nose

Teeth

Lips

Tongue

◀ **On the scent.** Your nose is always at work, helping you to breathe. But if you really want to *smell* something, you sniff hard. Sniffing sucks odors from the air up into your nose. The odors, which are tiny particles, land on skin that lines the top of the nostril. There a liquid called mucus keeps the inside of your nostrils moist. (Mucus is what comes out of your nose when you blow it or sneeze.) The tiny particles get trapped in the mucus, where nerve endings record the smell and send a message to your brain. As soon as the message reaches your brain, you know what the smell is.

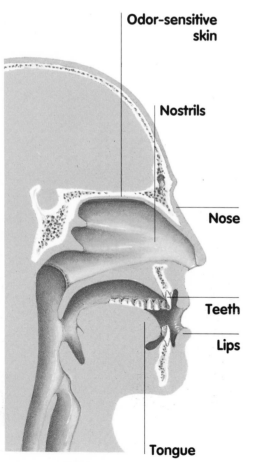

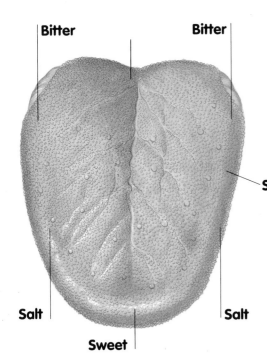

Bitter   Bitter

Salt   Salt

Sweet

Sour

◀ These are the areas of your tongue that sense different flavors of food. Your tongue also tells you if a food is hot or cold, or rough or smooth. When your taste buds detect the flavor in the food, they send a message to your brain, telling it what the food is.

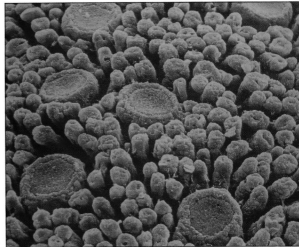

Surface of the tongue
(x 100)

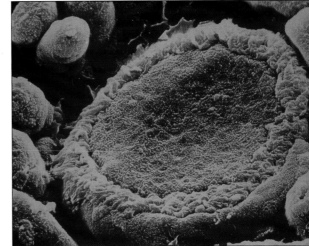

Taste bud
(x 2,000)

▶ **On the tip of your tongue.** Different parts of your tongue are sensitive to different tastes because your tongue has many tiny bumps on it called taste buds. These tell you if a food is salty, sweet, sour, or bitter. Some foods are mixtures of them all. Check which part of your tongue responds to each taste by testing different places on its surface with salt, sugar, lemon juice, and vinegar.

Now try putting food in your mouth and holding your nose as you eat. Because your sense of smell is cut off, you may find that you can't taste things very well.

Careful brushwork

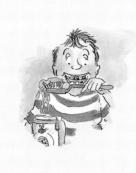

On the outside of your teeth is a hard coating called enamel. Acids or bacteria in the food you eat may attack the enamel and make holes in it called cavities. Sticky, sugary food and drinks are most likely to damage enamel, but correct brushing will clean off food and prevent cavities from forming.

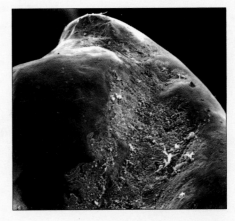

Tooth enamel
(x 25)

VITAL VISION

L ike little video cameras, your eyes take in and process an endless stream of color images every second that you are awake. Actually your eyes don't "see" at all. Instead they send electrical signals to your brain, which translates the signals into messages and recognizes the pictures. Each eye is packed with millions of special cells and lots of tiny, delicate muscles that help it to perform this difficult task.

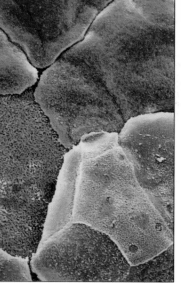

Cornea
(x 1,300)

▲ The tough, curved cornea is made up of many tiny cells. Because it is transparent, light can pass through it and reach the retina.

▼ **Seeing eye to eye.** The human eye is a round ball about an inch across. It is full of clear liquid and is partially covered by a transparent sheet called the cornea. The colored part is called the iris. The black circle in the middle, the pupil, is a hole in the eyeball. Behind it is a lens that directs light going through the iris onto the back of the eyeball. Here light-sensitive cells, packed into an area called the retina, record light and colors as chemical signals and send them along a special nerve pathway to the brain.

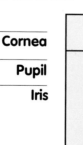

Nerve to brain

Muscles

Retina

Cornea

Pupil

Iris

Lens

Iris and pupil area of eyeball

DID YOU KNOW?

Your eyelashes and eyelids protect your eyes by preventing little bits of dirt and dust in the air from getting inside. Under your eyelids are special glands that make tears to wash away the particles that do manage to get in.

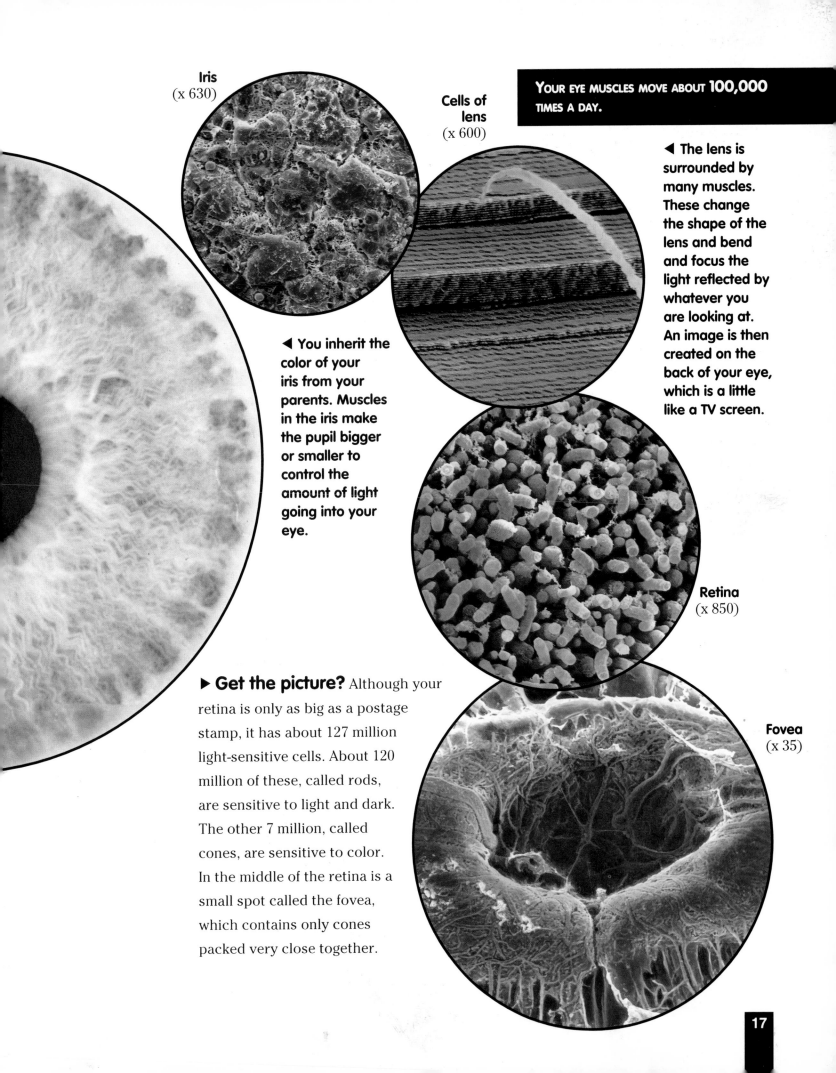

Iris
(x 630)

Cells of lens
(x 600)

◄ The lens is surrounded by many muscles. These change the shape of the lens and bend and focus the light reflected by whatever you are looking at. An image is then created on the back of your eye, which is a little like a TV screen.

◄ You inherit the color of your iris from your parents. Muscles in the iris make the pupil bigger or smaller to control the amount of light going into your eye.

Retina
(x 850)

Fovea
(x 35)

▶ **Get the picture?** Although your retina is only as big as a postage stamp, it has about 127 million light-sensitive cells. About 120 million of these, called rods, are sensitive to light and dark. The other 7 million, called cones, are sensitive to color. In the middle of the retina is a small spot called the fovea, which contains only cones packed very close together.

PLAY IT BY EAR

On the outside of your head are two oddly shaped flaps of skin—your ears. You can't move them around much, the way most animals can, but they do help you to hear sounds coming from all directions. The most important parts of your ears are inside your head. Besides enabling you to hear, your inner ears also help you to keep your balance as you move about.

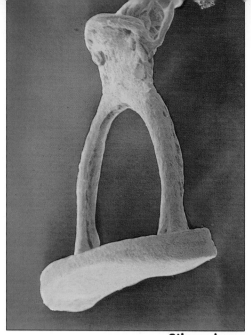

Stirrup bone
(x 40)

▲ The stirrup bone in your middle ear gets its name from its shape. It looks just like a stirrup used in horseback riding. The stirrup picks up vibrations from the eardrum and passes them on to the cochlea.

▼ **Sound system.** Your ears have three parts. The first is the hole you can stick your finger in, called the ear canal. At the end of this is a thin layer of skin called the eardrum. The next part, the middle ear, has three small bones and a structure called the eustachian tube, which leads to your throat and helps control the air pressure in your ear. The last part, the inner ear, has many sound-sensitive cells.

Every sound you hear causes air vibrations called sound waves. When sound waves reach your eardrum, they cause it to vibrate, thereby passing the sound on to your inner ear. A chemical signal generated by your inner ear is then sent to your brain, which processes it so you can "hear," or recognize, the sound.

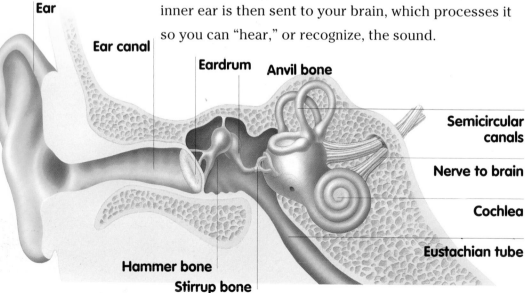

Ear

Ear canal

Eardrum   Anvil bone

Semicircular canals

Nerve to brain

Cochlea

Eustachian tube

Hammer bone

Stirrup bone

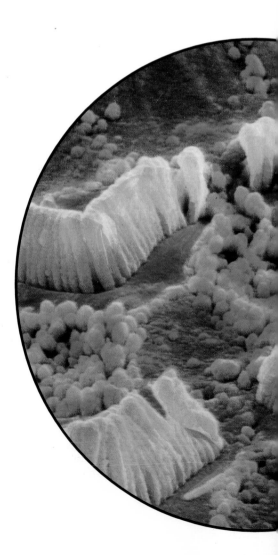

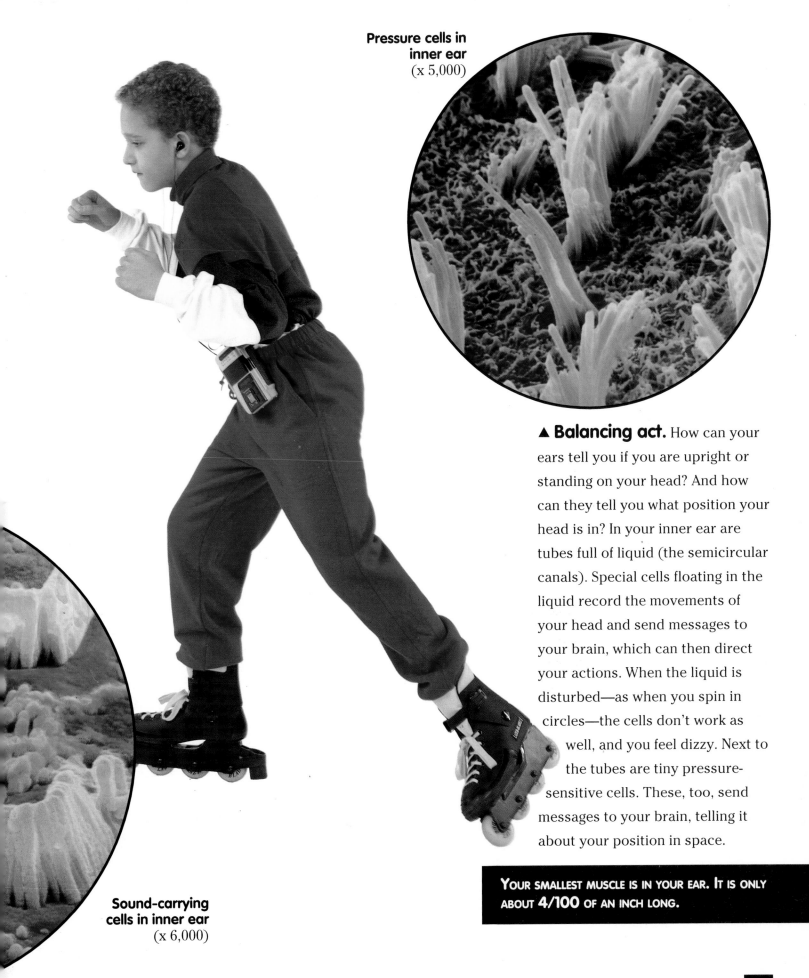

Pressure cells in inner ear
(x 5,000)

Sound-carrying cells in inner ear
(x 6,000)

▲ **Balancing act.** How can your ears tell you if you are upright or standing on your head? And how can they tell you what position your head is in? In your inner ear are tubes full of liquid (the semicircular canals). Special cells floating in the liquid record the movements of your head and send messages to your brain, which can then direct your actions. When the liquid is disturbed—as when you spin in circles—the cells don't work as well, and you feel dizzy. Next to the tubes are tiny pressure-sensitive cells. These, too, send messages to your brain, telling it about your position in space.

YOUR SMALLEST MUSCLE IS IN YOUR EAR. IT IS ONLY ABOUT **4/100** OF AN INCH LONG.

LIFE SUPPORT

Without your bones, you would be a big floppy bag of skin that couldn't move. Your skeleton has two main parts. The first is a central frame made up of your skull, backbone, shoulders, chest, and hips. This frame supports your body and gives you your shape. It also protects and supports the delicate organs inside. Your arm and leg bones make up the rest of your skeleton and let you move around. Your bones also manufacture blood cells and store useful minerals.

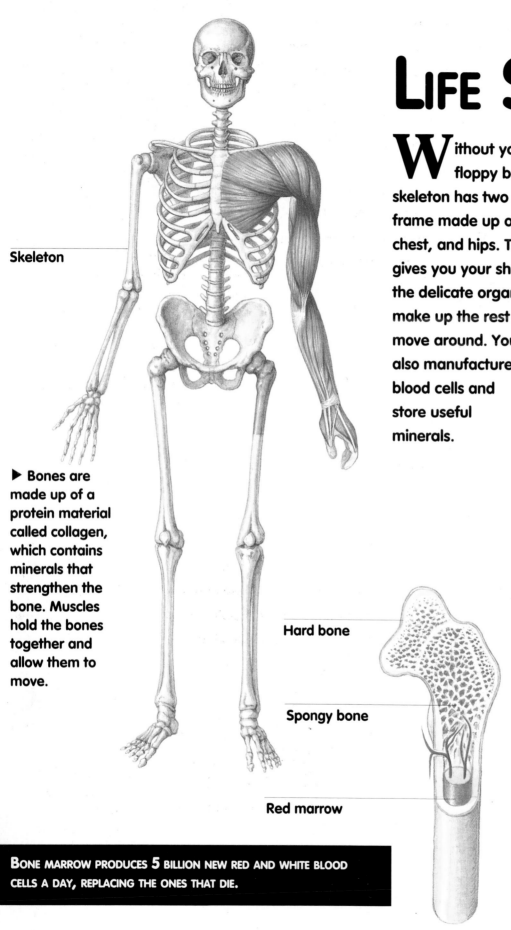

Skeleton

▶ Bones are made up of a protein material called collagen, which contains minerals that strengthen the bone. Muscles hold the bones together and allow them to move.

Hard bone

Spongy bone

Red marrow

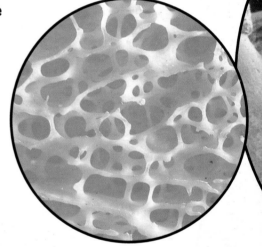

Spongy bone

BONE MARROW PRODUCES **5** BILLION NEW RED AND WHITE BLOOD CELLS A DAY, REPLACING THE ONES THAT DIE.

DID YOU KNOW?

When you were born, you had over 800 bones. As you grew, some of the bones in your skull and elsewhere joined together. When you are an adult, you will have 206 bones altogether—about half of them in your hands and feet.

▼ Close to the bone. A human thigh bone has a thick, hard outer shell. Inside the bone, at each end, is a network of fine rods called spongy bone. This arrangement makes the bone strong but light, able to support the body and help it move about.

The spaces between the rods of bone are filled with soft red bone marrow that makes new red and white blood cells. Some marrow also stores fat, which can be used when the body needs it.

Blood vessels go through channels in the bone. The blood brings the bone the nutrients it needs to grow and renew itself and takes away any waste material.

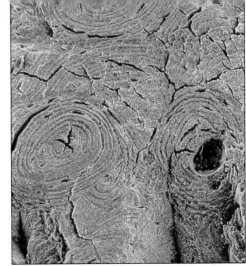

Compact bone
(x 140)

▲ Compact bone is the thick, strong outer layer of bone. This cross-section of a thigh bone shows the rings of bone surrounded by blood vessels and nerves. Blood carries minerals, such as phosphorus and calcium, to the bones. But the bones will give up the minerals if the body needs them somewhere else.

Spongy bone
(x 65)

Muscle

Bundle of fibers

Myofibril

▶ Muscle power. Muscles in the body attached to bones are called skeletal muscles. These bundles of fibers made of overlapping threads of protein come in two kinds, thick and thin. Each individual fiber is called a myofibril.

Chemical signals sent by the brain along the nerves cause the protein threads in the muscle fibers to move closer together. This shortens the muscle and makes it move.

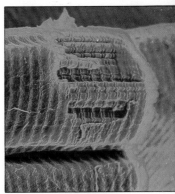

Myofibril
(x 1,200)

▲ A myofibril is the tiniest fiber that can be separated from a bundle of muscle.

AIR TIME

Take a deep breath. Now let it out. Most of the time you don't notice that you are doing these two basic things. Nor do you notice that your chest is moving gently up and down and that your two lungs are pumping away, taking in air and blowing it out again. Controlled by your brain, the muscles of your body work automatically so that you can breathe without having to think about it. You also use the air in your lungs to breathe out when you speak, sing, shout, or blow up a balloon.

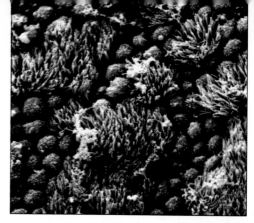

Hairs, or cilia, in breathing tubes
(x 1,000)

▲ The tubes leading to your lungs are lined with tiny hairs called cilia. These help to clean the air going into your lungs, collecting dust and other tiny particles.

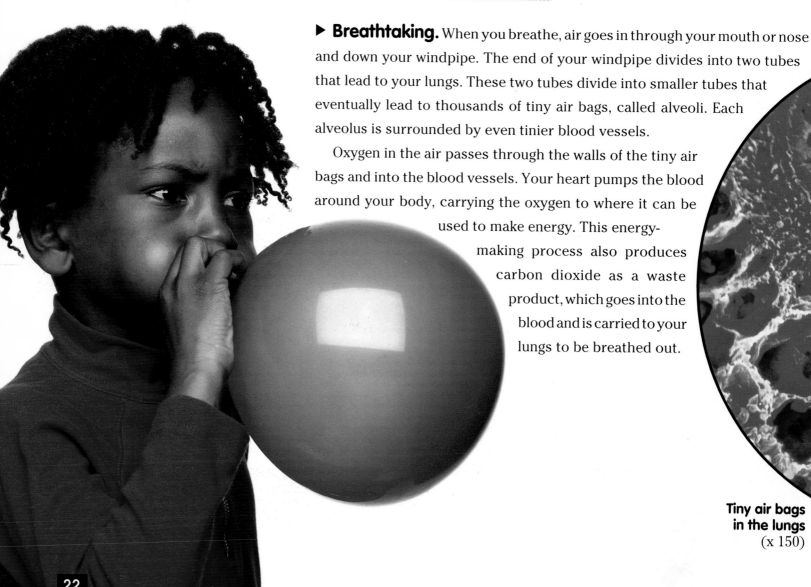

▶ **Breathtaking.** When you breathe, air goes in through your mouth or nose and down your windpipe. The end of your windpipe divides into two tubes that lead to your lungs. These two tubes divide into smaller tubes that eventually lead to thousands of tiny air bags, called alveoli. Each alveolus is surrounded by even tinier blood vessels.

Oxygen in the air passes through the walls of the tiny air bags and into the blood vessels. Your heart pumps the blood around your body, carrying the oxygen to where it can be used to make energy. This energy-making process also produces carbon dioxide as a waste product, which goes into the blood and is carried to your lungs to be breathed out.

**Tiny air bags
in the lungs**
(x 150)

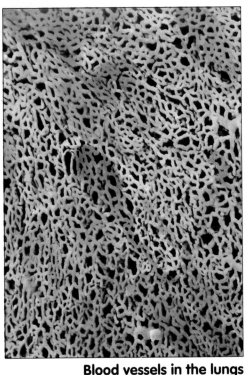

Blood vessels in the lungs
(x 160)

◀ Surrounding the walls of the tiny air bags in your lungs are millions of even tinier blood vessels. If these were all laid end to end, they would reach more than halfway around the world.

▶ Your windpipe (also called the trachea) is the primary tube of your breathing system. It leads to your two lungs, which then lead to the tiny air bags known as the alveoli.

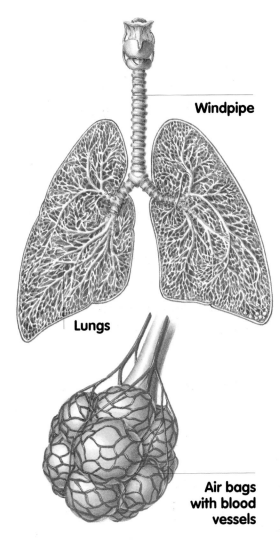

Windpipe

Lungs

Air bags with blood vessels

Pump it up. Muscles between your rib bones move the ribs up and down to pump air in and out of your lungs. When you take a deep breath, you can feel your chest swell outward and grow larger. There is also a big muscle called the diaphragm just under your ribs and above your stomach. This muscle moves down to draw air into your lungs and then moves up again to push the air out.

When you are sitting down or asleep, you breathe in and out about 18 times a minute. But when you run or play sports, you use more energy. Special chemicals in your blood send a message to your brain. Your brain sends the message to your muscles, and you breathe more quickly or pant. Your lungs take in more air, passing more oxygen to your body's cells and generating the energy you need.

DID YOU KNOW?

Your lungs hold enough air to fill a large balloon. Every time you breathe in, you take in about two cups' worth of air, which you make an effort to breathe out again. Even when you breathe out very hard, though, there is still a lot of air left in your lungs.

AN ADULT MALE RUNNING FAST BREATHES IN OVER **5** GALLONS OF AIR A MINUTE.

FOOD FACTORY

Where do you get the energy you need to play, sit still, or even breathe? Most of it comes from the food you eat and the liquids you drink. Your body also needs energy to grow, to get better when you are sick, to make new blood cells, and to do many other things. Before food can be used by your body, however, it has to go through your mouth, stomach, and intestines. This is called digestion.

▼ As soon as you bite into an apple (or any other food), your body starts to work on it. As you chew, saliva in your mouth begins to break down the food.

▶ **Chewing it over.** Chewed food is pushed by your tongue to the back of your mouth and down your food pipe, or esophagus. Here muscles squeeze together and push the food down into your stomach, where it stays for about three hours. Muscles in your stomach walls churn the food, breaking it down into a pulp and mixing it with strong chemical juices. The juices turn the pulp into substances that can be absorbed by the body later.

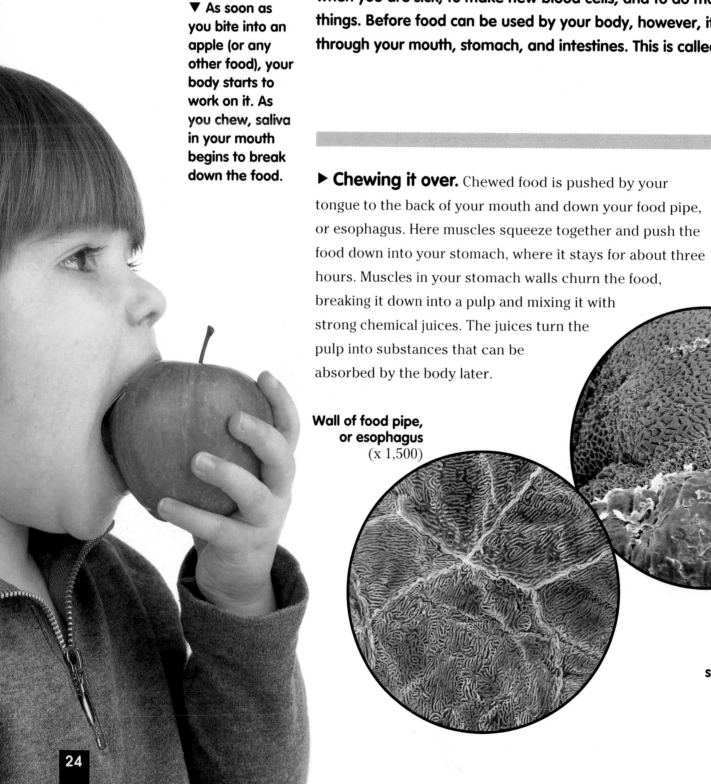

Wall of food pipe, or esophagus
(x 1,500)

End of esophagus (*purple*) and beginning of stomach (*green*)
(x 100)

▼ Villi along the wall of the small intestine absorb nutrients from the food as they bathe in the liquidy food pulp.

Wall of small intestine where it joins large intestine (x 120)

Villi (x 80)

Juice gland from wall of stomach (x 850)

▶ These are the important parts of your digestive system, which is almost 33 feet long. It takes about 24 hours from eating to eliminating solid waste from the body.

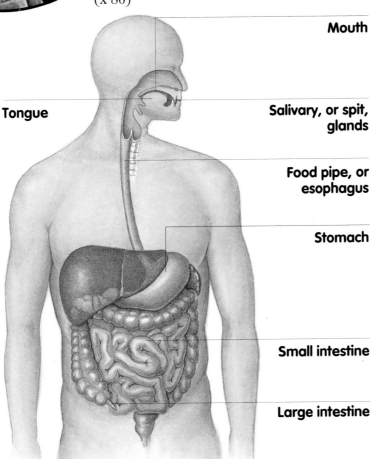

Mouth

Tongue

Salivary, or spit, glands

Food pipe, or esophagus

Stomach

Small intestine

Large intestine

◀ **Facts to digest.** Food pulp in your stomach moves a little at a time into your small intestine, a very long tube coiled below your stomach. Additional juices secreted by glands and by the walls of the small intestine mix with the pulp to further break it down, or digest it. Thousands of tiny fingerlike structures called villi line the small intestine. The digested food goes through the villi into the bloodstream. What is left—the tough, woody parts that can't be digested—goes into the large intestine, where it later exits your body as waste.

DID YOU KNOW?

Your stomach muscles sometimes keep moving even after all the food you have eaten has been passed on to your small intestine. This gives you the sensation of hunger pains. Hunger pains stop as soon as you eat something again.

25

ALL IN THE BLOOD

Blood is your internal transportation system and is a very important part of the breathing process. It carries food and oxygen to every part of your body except the nails, hair, and front of the eyes. It also helps keep the body at just the right temperature, fights off germs and diseases, and forms scabs to stop wounds from bleeding.

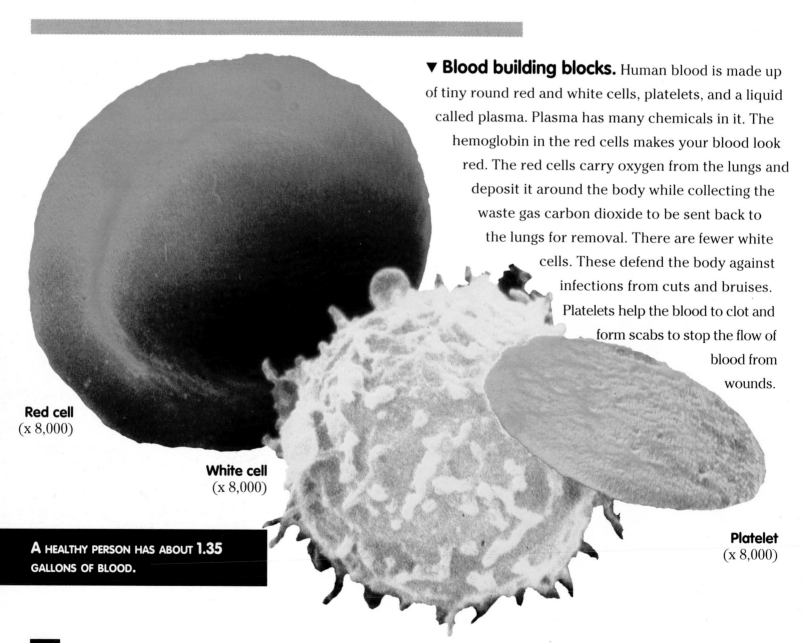

▼ **Blood building blocks.** Human blood is made up of tiny round red and white cells, platelets, and a liquid called plasma. Plasma has many chemicals in it. The hemoglobin in the red cells makes your blood look red. The red cells carry oxygen from the lungs and deposit it around the body while collecting the waste gas carbon dioxide to be sent back to the lungs for removal. There are fewer white cells. These defend the body against infections from cuts and bruises. Platelets help the blood to clot and form scabs to stop the flow of blood from wounds.

Red cell
(x 8,000)

White cell
(x 8,000)

Platelet
(x 8,000)

A HEALTHY PERSON HAS ABOUT 1.35 GALLONS OF BLOOD.

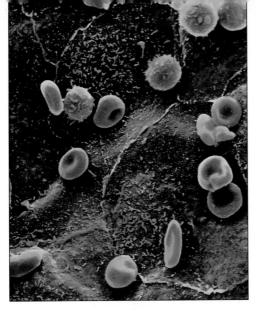

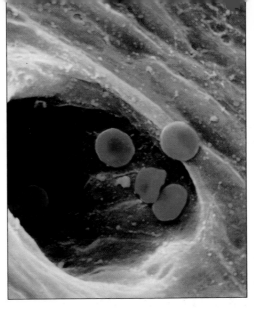

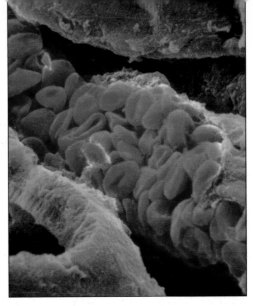

Red cells inside the heart
(x 1,000)

Red cells moving from large artery into small one
(x 1,000)

Red cells in tiny blood vessel
(x 1,000)

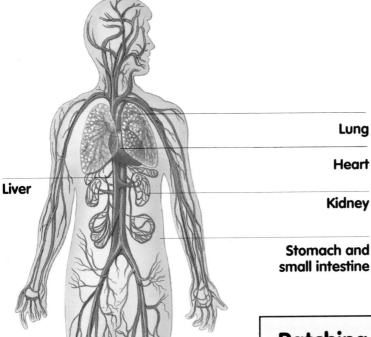

Lung

Heart

Kidney

Liver

Stomach and small intestine

Circulation of blood

◄ **Mobile blood.** Blood is pumped around the body by the heart. First, oxygen from the lungs is picked up by the blood and carried along large blood vessels called arteries. The arteries divide into smaller and smaller vessels, right down to tiny capillaries. After the blood has delivered its oxygen to sites that need it, it picks up carbon dioxide from the body and returns it to the lungs via vessels called veins. Once there, the blood collects more oxygen. Blood also delivers chemicals and digested food substances from the intestines to all parts of the body and takes away waste.

Patching up

When your skin gets cut, blood may ooze from the wound and germs can enter your body. To heal the wound, the platelets in your blood work together with a special substance called fibrin (seen here on a red blood cell) to make the blood clot and form a scab over the wound.

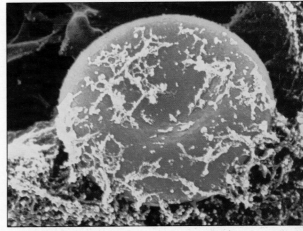

Red blood cell covered with fibrin (x 6,000)

GETTING THE MESSAGE

Is there really complex electrical circuitry inside your body? Believe it or not, this is exactly what your nerves, brain, and spinal column really are. Your nervous system helps keep you alive by telling you what is going on outside as well as inside your body. It works by electrical signals shooting through billions of nerve cells every second, passing on information and instructions.

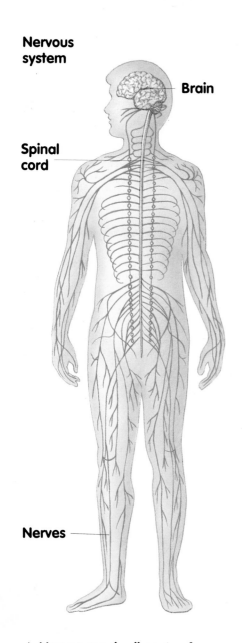

Nervous system

Brain

Spinal cord

Nerves

▲ Nerves reach all parts of your body. The most important ones are connected to your brain, which receives information and sends back instructions.

▶ **Plenty of nerve.** Your body has three main types of nerve cells. One type receives information from your senses, which tell you about the things you smell, taste, see, hear, and feel. These nerve cells send the information to your brain and to other parts of your nervous system.

The second type of nerve cells carries messages from your nervous system to your muscles and glands, telling them what to do. They keep your heart beating, your lungs breathing, your eyelids blinking, and all the other parts of your body working. The third type are the linking nerves, which shuttle messages from one cell to the next, using electrical impulses.

▶ Inside your backbone is your spinal cord, which is made up of bundles of nerve cells that carry messages to and from your brain.

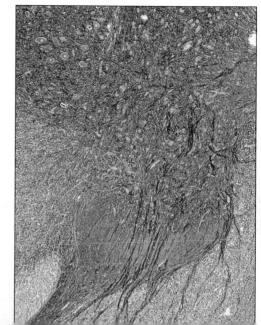

Spinal cord
(x 80)

▼ **Nerve center.** Your brain contains masses of nerve cells. Some are message receivers and some are message senders. The simplest reaction to a message is one that bypasses your brain entirely—you don't think about it at all. If you touch something very hot, you immediately pull your hand away. This is because the nerves in your fingertips have alerted your nervous system that your fingers are in danger. Your muscles get the message, and your hand quickly moves away from the heat so your fingers don't get burned. This is a reflex action.

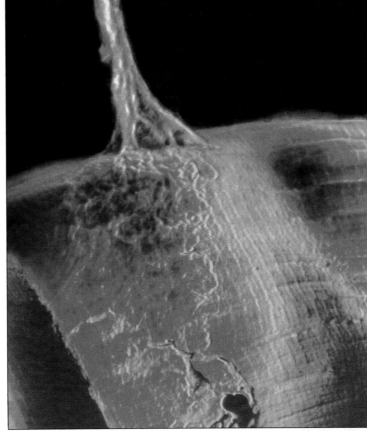

Nerve cell joined to muscle
(x 700)

Bundles of linking cells

Nerve cell

Muscles

Brain nerve cells
(x 230)

▲ When a message from your fingertips reaches the nerve cells joined to the muscles in your arm, the muscles contract. This pulls your hand quickly away from the heat.

Kerchoo!

Sneezing is a reflex action. When something irritating like dust or pepper settles on the nerve endings in your nose, it makes you take a deep breath. The top of your windpipe closes, and the pressure builds up in your lungs. Then your windpipe opens again and the air explodes out in a sneeze, blowing the dust or pepper out of your nose.

How Life Begins

Every human baby starts out as a tiny egg inside its mother. But the egg can only grow and develop into a baby after a sperm from the father fertilizes, or joins together with, the egg. When this happens, the sperm and the egg become one cell. That cell contains the genetic blueprints—skin color, hair color, and eye color, as well as the other things that are special to any one human being—passed along by its father and mother. The father's sperm determines what sex the baby will be.

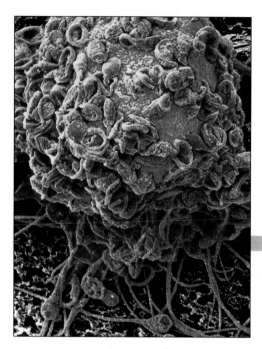

Sperm on egg
(x 700)

◀ **Sperm are like tiny tadpoles with long tails. Hundreds of them will swarm over an egg, trying to get inside and fertilize it. As soon as the egg lets one in, its surface thickens to keep out all the other sperm, which soon die.**

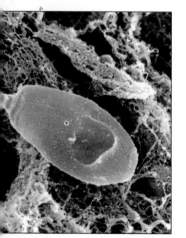

Sperm
(x 4,500)

▶ **The great divide.** One day or so after fertilization the egg divides into two cells. During the next few days, it divides into still more cells. The egg is then smaller than a pencil point but will keep growing for the next nine months. As it grows, a sac develops around it, and it floats in a bag of protective liquid. After about three weeks, the heart starts beating.

With a special cord, this tiny blob of new life called an embryo is linked to its mother's blood supply. It gets food and oxygen from her blood. Soon the embryo has a head, a brain, and a spine. At two months the embryo is called a fetus—and later a baby.

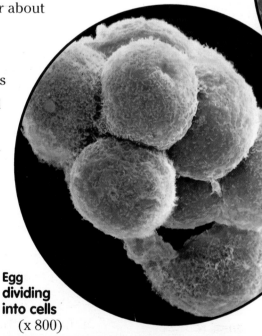

Egg dividing into cells
(x 800)

AT ABOUT SIX MONTHS A FETUS CAN HEAR AND WILL EVEN JUMP AT VERY SUDDEN LOUD NOISES.

▼ At seven weeks the embryo is about the size of a small walnut. Its legs have begun to grow, and its fingers and toes can be seen.

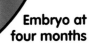

Embryo at four months

Embryo at seven weeks

Embryo at five weeks

▲ After about five weeks, the embryo's head starts to take shape. The dark spot is an eye. The arms and legs look like buds, and the small red spot is its heart.

Growth spurt. By four months (*above right*) the fetus is beginning to look very much like a baby. The arms and hands are almost fully developed, and so are the legs and feet. The ears have developed, and the eyes are in position but do not yet have eyelids.

At seven months the fetus weighs a little over 2 pounds. It is now moving around, kicking its legs and waving its arms.

At nine months the baby weighs from about 6 to 8 pounds. Shortly before the baby is ready to be born, the bag of special liquid surrounding it breaks. At birth the baby starts to breathe, and the cord that joined it to its mother is cut.

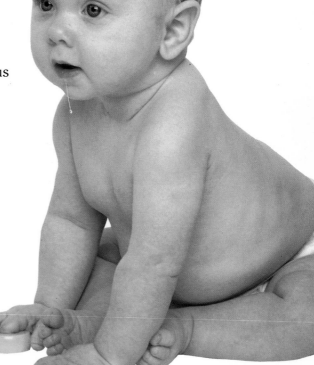

THE BODY AT WAR

How do people get sick? Like soldiers in an army, tiny bacteria and viruses can invade the human body and make a person ill. They enter the body through the mouth and nose when we breathe, through scratches, cuts, and insect bites, and through the food we eat. A healthy body can usually fight off most diseases by itself, but sometimes medicine or surgery is needed to make a person well again.

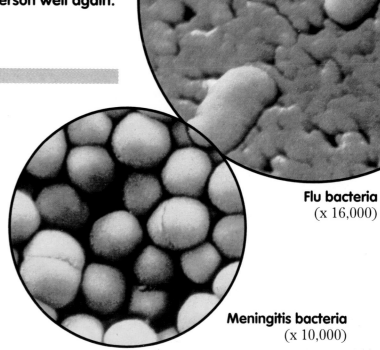

Flu bacteria
(x 16,000)

Meningitis bacteria
(x 10,000)

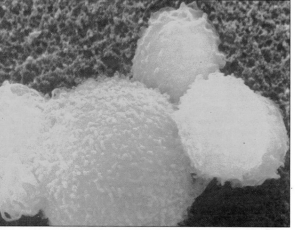

◀ **White blood cells help fight disease. These four white cells are attacking a cancerous growth called a tumor.**

White blood cells attacking tumor
(x 4,500)

VIRUSES CAUSE DISEASES SUCH AS **AIDS** AND THE FLU, NEITHER OF WHICH HAS A CURE.

◀ **Defenseless.** The white blood cell to the left is being attacked by the human immunodeficiency virus (HIV), which causes AIDS. The virus (shown here as green dots) will continue to multiply and eventually destroy the cell. Later the virus will spread to more cells, killing them as well. In time so many cells will be destroyed that the person's body will no longer be able to fight off other infections.

◀ **HIV virus on white blood cell**
(x 7,000)

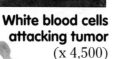

◀ These rodlike bacteria cause a type of bacterial flu. Flu is more often caused by a virus. The round bacteria *(lower left)* cause meningitis, a brain infection.

Tuberculosis bacteria (x 5,000)

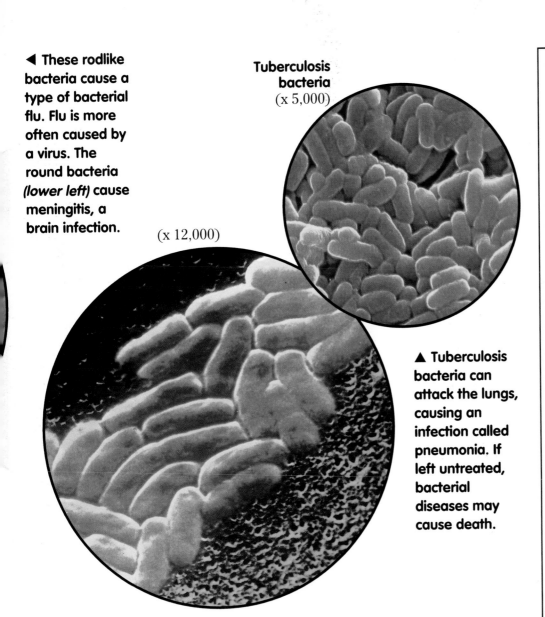

(x 12,000)

▲ Tuberculosis bacteria can attack the lungs, causing an infection called pneumonia. If left untreated, bacterial diseases may cause death.

Fighting fire with fire? Today one of the main weapons in the fight against disease is vaccination. A person, usually a child, gets a shot or drinks a liquid that contains some of the germs that cause a disease. The germs have been killed or weakened by special methods. The body's defense system can easily fight off these germs and at the same time build up protection, called antibodies, against that particular disease. If a person later comes into contact with the germs of the real disease, his or her antibodies will fight off the germs and the person won't become sick. Vaccinations are given to prevent such diseases as whooping cough, diphtheria, mumps, and measles.

Dainty needlework

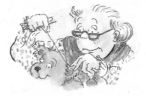

Microsurgery is an amazing form of modern surgery in which tiny, delicate instruments are used and doctors watch what they are doing on a television screen hooked up to a microscope. A surgeon's needle may only be as long as this hyphen (-). The doctor below is performing eye surgery.

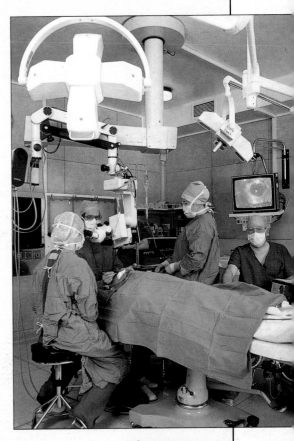

Microsurgery

PEOPLE PESTS

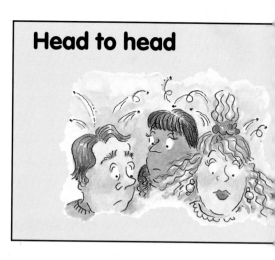

People are never alone, even when they think they are. That's because millions of tiny creatures are living in or on their bodies. Some just visit for a quick meal, but others "move in"—spending their whole lives with a human "host." They can make a person feel itchy. Though most do not cause serious illnesses, some can transmit diseases from one person to another.

Fungus of athlete's foot
(x 2,000)

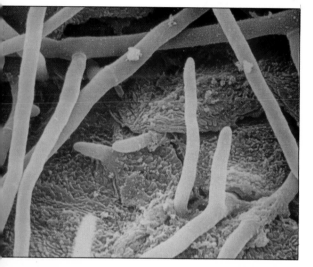

Athlete's foot

▼ The sore, cracked skin on the foot below was caused by the athlete's foot fungus.

Fungus foot. Athlete's foot is an infection caused by a fungus that can be picked up very easily in warm, damp places, such as locker rooms. Some people have such a mild infection that they don't even know it is there. If the infection is severe, the skin on the feet is itchy and can become scaly and blistered, particularly between the toes. Keeping the feet dry and well dusted with talcum powder and changing socks every day usually gets rid of the fungus. Creams that kill the fungus may be prescribed by a doctor if the infection persists.

DID YOU KNOW?

Millions of tiny bacteria live on human skin without doing any harm. The warm, moist skin of a human armpit contains as many as 500 bacteria in an area the size of the period at the end of this sentence.

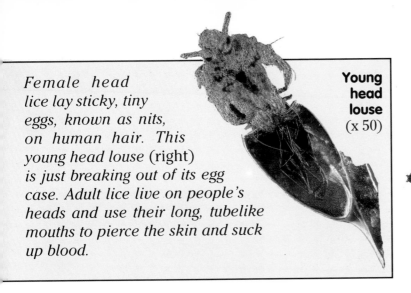

Female head lice lay sticky, tiny eggs, known as nits, on human hair. This young head louse (right) is just breaking out of its egg case. Adult lice live on people's heads and use their long, tubelike mouths to pierce the skin and suck up blood.

Young head louse (x 50)

Body louse (x 70)

▲ Body lice live in the seams and folds of people's clothes. They feed on a person's blood and make the skin sore and itchy. These lice may also spread diseases.

▼ **Blood banquet.** Female mosquitoes land on human skin and use their tubelike mouths to suck up blood. In hot climates some mosquitoes carry thousands of tiny parasites that cause the disease malaria. When a mosquito bites someone, the parasites pass through the wound into the blood. They rapidly multiply in the red blood cells. Sometimes they burst out of the blood cells and cause the person to have an attack of malaria.

The mosquito seen here lives in cold northern climates. It does not carry malaria, but its bite can cause a large, itchy lump on a person's skin.

Head of mosquito (x 25)

Mosquito on skin

EACH YEAR OVER **200** MILLION PEOPLE LIVING IN THE TROPICS CATCH MALARIA, AND **2** MILLION DIE FROM IT.

GUESS WHAT?

Read the clues, then try to guess what these images are. You'll find the answers at the bottom of the page.

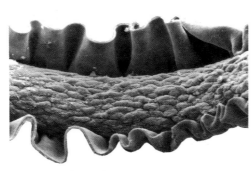

1. Mysterious cave? You could only explore this place if someone gobbled you up!

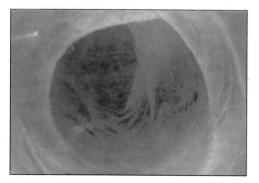

2. A snake shedding its skin? It's okay to tangle with this, because it's totally harmless.

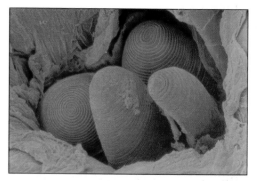

3. Worm babies? Brand-new yet already dead, these still grow very quickly.

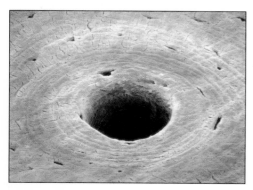

4. Hole in one? You'd feel a bit below par if you broke one of these.

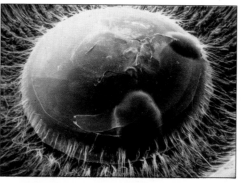

5. Gigantic jellyfish? You're using two of these as you try to recognize this picture.

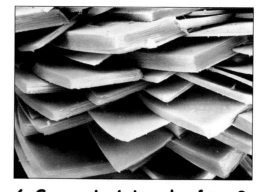

6. Carpenter's two-by-fours? These are certainly essential parts of your basic framework.

7. Pasta salad? Don't be tempted—even a little bit would be very bad for your health.

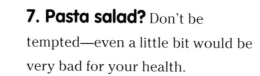

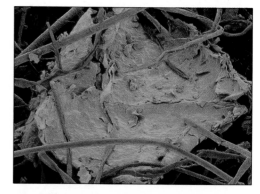

8. Gift wrap with streamers? This wraps *you* up from head to toe.

GLOSSARY

Alveoli — the tiny air bags in the lungs. Oxygen passes through the walls of these air bags into the blood vessels.

Cilia — tiny hairs that line the tubes leading to the lungs. Cilia help clean the air going into your lungs. Your nose also has cilia in it, which stimulate odor-sensitive cells to send messages to the brain.

Cornea — the tough, curved cover at the front of the eye. It is clear so that light can go right through it into the eye.

Diaphragm — the large muscle just under your ribs that moves down to draw air into your lungs and up again to push the air out.

Digestion — a series of processes that take place in your mouth, stomach, and intestines to break down food into different substances. Your body then uses these substances to make energy.

Eardrum — the thin layer of skin in the ear that vibrates when sound waves reach it. The eardrum passes on the vibrations to other parts of the ear.

Embryo — a baby at an early stage of development inside its mother.

Fovea — a small spot in the middle of the retina of the eye. It contains masses of color-sensitive cells that help you see things in great detail.

Iris — the colored part of the eye. Its muscles alter the size of the pupil and control the amount of light going into the eye.

Keratin — the tough material that makes up hair and nails.

Lens — the rounded transparent structure behind the iris of the eye that helps you focus.

Nerve cells — cells throughout the body that carry or transmit messages to and from the brain.

Nervous system — the combination of nerves, the brain, and the spinal cord that passes information and instructions around the body to keep it working.

Platelets — tiny cells in the blood that help it to clot.

Pupil — the black circle, which is a hole, in the middle of the eye. The pupil allows light to enter the eye.

Red blood cells — cells in the blood that carry oxygen from the lungs to the rest of the body. They also take back waste gas.

Retina — the area at the back of the eye that is packed with special light-sensitive cells. The retina detects light and colors, records them as pictures, and sends them as messages to the brain.

Skeleton — the framework of bones that supports your body and protects the delicate parts inside.

Skin — the tough, waterproof cover all over your body. Skin is full of blood vessels and nerves. It also contains hair roots and sweat glands.

Spinal cord — bundles of nerve cells inside the backbone, which carry messages to and from your brain.

Taste buds — cells on your tongue that detect the flavor of food and send a message to the brain telling you what each taste is.

Villi — tiny, fingerlike projections that line the small intestine. The villi help digested food to be absorbed into the bloodstream.

White blood cells — cells in the blood that help protect the body from disease and repair parts that are damaged.

INDEX

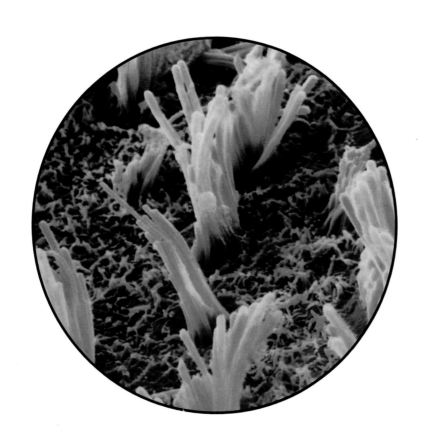

The authors and publishers would like to thank Andrew Syred of Microscopix, Liz Hirst at the National Institute of Medical Research, and Steve Gorton for their assistance in the preparation of this book, as well as the other photographers and organizations listed below for their kind permission to reproduce the following photographs:

Dr. Tony Brain: 6 top right, 7 top right, 10 left of center, 13 bottom right, 15 bottom right, 22 top right, 35 top right, back cover right of center

Steve Gorton: 6-7, 9 bottom, 10 bottom, 12 left, 13 right, 14-15 bottom, 19 left, 22 bottom left, 24 bottom left, 29 bottom left, 31 bottom right

The Natural History Museum, London: 36 above center

Science Photo Library: 13 top left and left of center; **Biophoto Associates**: 34 top; **Dr. Tony Brain**: 11 left of center, 13 above center; **Jeremy Burgess**: 7 left of center and right of center, 9 top right and right of center; **CNRI**: 3 right of center, 10 right of center, 18 top right, 21 top right and bottom right, 22-23 bottom, 27 top right, 28-29 center, 32 top right and center, 33 above center and left, 36 bottom left; **A. B. Dowsett**: 27 bottom right; **Ralph Eagle**: front cover center, 16-17 center, 36 center; **Stevie Grand**: 4 bottom left; **Manfred Kage**: 35 center and 36 top left; **Dr. Andrejs Liepins**: 32 left of center; **Dr. P. Marazzi**: 34 bottom; **Professor P. Motta**, Dept. of Anatomy, University of "La Sapienza", Rome: 3 left, 5 left and right, 8-9 top, 16 top left, 17 top left, top right, right of center, and bottom right, 18-19 bottom, 19 top right, 20-21, 23 top left, 24 below center and bottom right, 25 top left and top right, 27 top left and above center, 30 bottom left, 36 left of center and right of center, back cover top left; **Professors P. M. Motta, K. R. Porter**, and **P. M. Andrews**: 24-25 center; **Professors P. M. Motta and J. van Blerkon**: 30 bottom right; **NASA**: 1, 6 center; **NIBSC**: 26, 32 bottom left; **Claude Nurisdany and Marie Perennou**: 20 right; **OMIKRON**: 3 bottom right, 15 top right and right of center; **Petit Format/Nestlé**: 30-31 center, 31 center and top right, back cover bottom left; **J. C. Revy**: 35 top left; **St. Bartholomew's Hospital**: 33 bottom right; **David Scharf**: 10-11 center, 30 top left, 36 top right and bottom right; **SECCHI-LECAQUE, ROUSSEL-UCLAF, CNRI**: 14 top right, 29 top right; **Jeremy Trew**: 4 top left

Andrew Syred, Microscopix: 4 top right, right of center, bottom right, and below center, 11 top left and right*, 12 below center and right, 28 bottom right, 35 bottom right

ZEFA: front cover left and right

* Photograph specially hand-colored by Helen Z.

ILLUSTRATORS:

Richard Coombes: 20, 21, 27 left, 28
Jane Gedye: 6, 13, 15 bottom left, 27 bottom center, 29 bottom right, 33, 34
Paul Richardson: 8, 14, 15 top left, 23, 25
Ed Stuart: 5 center, 16, 18, 29 center

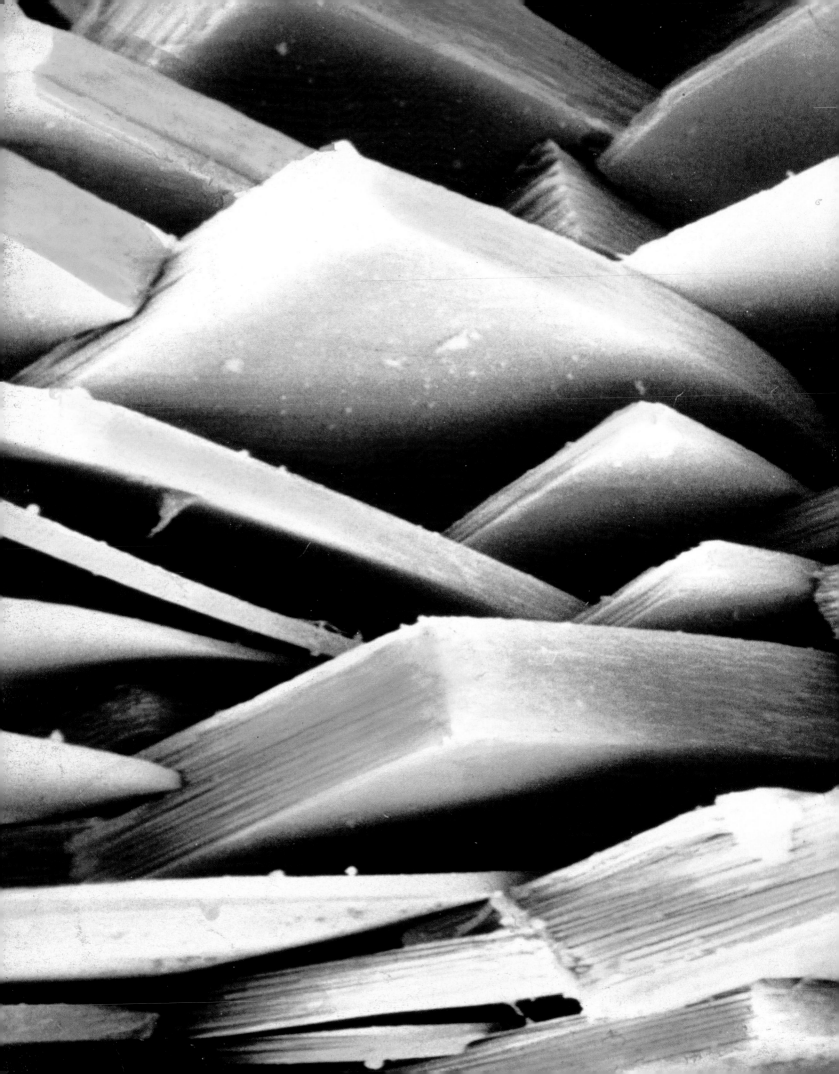

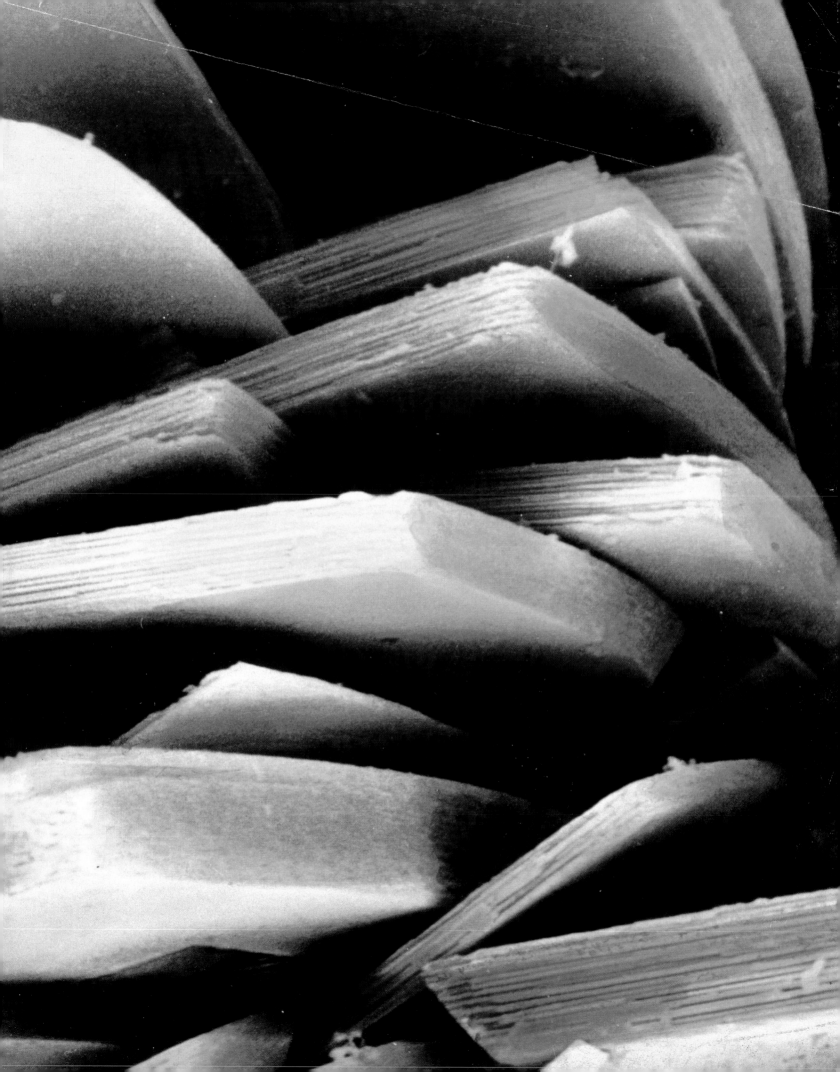